THE SILENT WARRIOR'S

Practical Communication Aid

A Partner Supported Resource for Neurogenic Communication Disorders

Brigette Foresman

Thank you for purchasing

The Silent Warrior's Practical Communication Aid.

Please inform others of this alternative communication aid and together we can help

~Break the Silence~

for those dealing with communications disorders.

Reviews are greatly appreciated and your opinion is very important to others searching for resource books to assist them with their family member, friend, or patient who has been diagnosed with a communication disorder.

Website: www.TheSilentWarriorBook.com

Thank you!

Brigette Foresman

Life's journey holds no guarantee

Of traveling a path without conflict-

Acknowledge, for no one, is immune-

Yet, within all of us, lies a silent warrior-

To engage the remaining journey with bravery-

-Brigette Foresman

The Silent Warrior's Practical Communication Aid book is for a person diagnosed with a medical condition resulting in the impairment of speech and the loss of mobility of his or hers arms/hands, to the extent of the inability to communicate through writing and or the use of technological communication devices.

The Silent Warrior book implements various topics & scenarios within a person's everyday routine, along with their adult responsibilities. It is of great importance for your family member and or patient to maintain as much control in the continuance of their life, as they now have to adapt and relearn to live with either a prolonged rehabilitation process or life-altering circumstance and your patience as a communication partner will help them find the bravery needed to move forward.

CONTENTS

Additional blank charts
available online:

TheSilentWarriorBook.com

~Communication Partner Guidelines~

This resource book is for a person experiencing a speech communication disorder and the loss of arm/hand mobility resulting in the inability to communicate through writing and or technological devices.

The following guidelines will assist an individual of any age, who can read, with communication between their family, friends, caregivers, and medical professionals.

- The communication partnership will consists of a "*Point-and-Signal*" method.
- Once your family member/patient has had their reading comprehension evaluated, you will need to establish the body signal for communication (see pg. 2 for examples). Whichever signal is used, one signal is for "No," and twice the signal is for "Yes."
- It would be helpful to place a quick reference communication board (e.g. small dry erase board or poster board) in the room to inform caregivers on rotation, family member, friends, and other guests to become familiar with the established signal for communication, along with the use of *The Silent Warrior's Practical Communication Aid*.
- Review the book's pages thoroughly with your family member/patient in order to become familiar with the set-up of the various topic pages (charts), with the listed phrases, questions, and responses.
- Begin with either the chart titled "Begin Here" on page 3 or the "Communication Topic Chart" on page 98- this is the simplified version of the topics listed in the contents.
- With each topic page, allow sufficient time for your family member/patient to glance over the page. Begin with this question, "Do you see a phrase on this page which will convey what you would like to communicate?" If the signal response is "No," look to see if that *topic* has more than one page of listed phrases, if it does not, proceed to using the Alphabet Chart as an alternate communication method.
- The row shown below is a sample of the top row printed on each topic chart, which will serve as a reminder for the communication partner to ask their family member/patient if they would like to use one of the *alternate communication charts* and to remember to "*ask or point*" to the top row, "**I DO NOT SEE A PHRASE I CAN USE.**"

I DO NOT SEE A PHRASE I CAN USE.	
LET'S USE THE ALPHABET CHART.	**LET'S USE THE TOPICS CHART.**

The pages within *The Silent Warrior's Practical Communication Aid* do not have double-sided printing in order to allow each individual to establish their own style of chart organization.

- **Communication partners may find it simpler to remove the pages from the book, and place them in sheet protectors or to have them laminated at your local office supply store and then reorganize the pages into a 3-ring binder or in a portable file box with each of the topics labeled on a file divider tab.**

This book will assist a person in need of communicating his or hers daily choices, decisions, needs, and responsibilities. It would be helpful to remove certain pages from this book that may cause emotional despair for your family member/patient, such as the section on nutrition- if your family member/patient is on a feeding tube, they do not need to see pages of food items they cannot eat.

Finding a way to adapt to the physical & emotional changes brought on by neurogenic communication disorders, neurological disorders, or a traumatic brain injury is one of life's most difficult healthcare occurrences. May the patients, along with their families, friends, and healthcare professionals find the strength from the silent warrior within each of them, to journey forward with patience and strength.

RIGHT HAND SQUEEZE	**RIGHT HAND FINGER/ THUMB TAP**	**RIGHT ARM OR HAND MOVEMENT**
LEFT HAND SQUEEZE	**LEFT HAND FINGER/ THUMB TAP**	**LEFT ARM OR HAND MOVEMENT**
EYE BLINK	**HEAD NOD**	**TONGUE EXTEND**
RIGHT FOOT OR LEG MOVEMENT	**LEFT FOOT OR LEG MOVEMENT**	**LIP SIGNAL**

LET'S USE THE
TOPICS CHART
PAGE 98

LET'S USE THE
SPOUSE/PARTNER
TOPICS CHART
PAGE 78

LET'S USE THE
ALPHABET CHART
PAGE 91

LET'S USE THE
PLANNER TOPICS CHART
PAGE 95

~HEAD~

I DO NOT SEE A PHRASE I CAN USE.			
LET'S USE THE ALPHABET CHART.		LET'S USE THE TOPICS CHART.	
I FEEL PRESSURE IN THE FRONT OF MY HEAD.	I HAVE A HEADACHE.	I HAVE A MIGRAINE.	I FEEL DIZZY WHEN SITTING.
I FEEL PRESSURE IN THE BACK OF MY HEAD.	MY HEAD FEELS HOT.	I WOULD LIKE AN ICE BAG ON MY HEAD.	I FEEL DIZZY WHEN STANDING.

4

~HEAD~

I DO NOT SEE A PHRASE I CAN USE.

LET'S USE THE ALPHABET CHART.

LET'S USE THE TOPICS CHART.

MY JAW HURTS ON THE

- RIGHT SIDE
- LEFT SIDE

I FEEL MUSCLE SPASMS IN MY FACE.

MY HEAD ITCHES.

MY JAW IS STIFF.

I HAVE A PAIN IN MY

- RIGHT CHEEK
- LEFT CHEEK

MY FACE FEELS DRY.

I HAVE PAIN IN BOTH SIDES OF MY FACE.

~EARS~

I DO NOT SEE A PHRASE I CAN USE.

LET'S USE THE ALPHABET CHART.	LET'S USE THE TOPICS CHART.

I CANNOT HEAR IN THE

- RIGHT EAR
- LEFT EAR
- BOTH EARS

I HAVE AN ITCH IN THE

- RIGHT EAR
- LEFT EAR
- BOTH EARS

I FEEL PAIN IN THE

- RIGHT EAR
- LEFT EAR
- BOTH EARS

IT FEELS LIKE I HAVE WATER IN THE

- RIGHT EAR
- LEFT EAR
- BOTH EARS

THERE IS A RINGING IN THE

- RIGHT EAR
- LEFT EAR
- BOTH EARS

PLEASE SWAB MY EARS.

I WOULD LIKE MY HEARING CHECKED.

~EYES~

I DO NOT SEE A PHRASE I CAN USE.

| LET'S USE THE ALPHABET CHART. | LET'S USE THE TOPICS CHART. |

I CANNOT SEE OUT OF MY

- RIGHT EYE
- LEFT EYE

MY EYES

- BURN
- FEEL DRY
- HURT
- ITCH

I SEE SPOTS IN MY

- RIGHT EYE
- LEFT EYE

I HAVE BLURRED VISION IN MY

- RIGHT EYE
- LEFT EYE

PLEASE PUT SOME EYE DROPS IN MY EYES.

I FEEL PRESSURE IN

- MY RIGHT EYE
- MY LEFT EYE
- BOTH EYES

7

~EYES~

I DO NOT SEE A PHRASE I CAN USE.	
LET'S USE THE ALPHABET CHART.	LET'S USE THE TOPICS CHART.

I NEED MY READING GLASSES.	I NEED MY PRESCRIPTION GLASSES.	I NEED TO MAKE AN APPOINTMENT WITH MY EYE DOCTOR.
PLEASE REMOVE MY GLASSES.	I WOULD LIKE MY CONTACTS PUT IN.	PLEASE CLEAN MY CONTACTS.
I WOULD LIKE TO WEAR MY SUNGLASSES.	PLEASE REMOVE MY CONTACTS.	I WOULD LIKE TO MAKE AN APPOINTMENT TO HAVE A VISION EXAM.

~MOUTH~

I DO NOT SEE A PHRASE I CAN USE.

LET'S USE THE ALPHABET CHART.

LET'S USE THE TOPICS CHART.

I BURNED MY TONGUE ON A HOT FOOD / BEVERAGE ITEM.

MY LIPS ARE

- CHAPPED
- TINGLING
- BURNING

I CANNOT TASTE ANYTHING.

MY TONGUE FEELS SWOLLEN.

MY MOUTH FEELS
- NUMB
- VERY DRY

MY LIPS FEEL SWOLLEN.

MY TONGUE HURTS.

THE INSIDE OF MY CHEEKS HURT.

I BIT MY TONGUE.

~MOUTH~

I DO NOT SEE A PHRASE I CAN USE.	
LET'S USE THE ALPHABET CHART.	LET'S USE THE TOPICS CHART.

I AM HAVING TROUBLE SWALLOWING.	THE ROOF OF MY MOUTH • HURTS • IS SWOLLEN	I HAVE A LOOSE TOOTH.
MY TEETH FEEL SENSITIVE.	MY GUMS HURT.	I THINK I HAVE LOST A FILLING.
I HAVE A TOOTHACHE.	I WOULD LIKE AN OVER-THE-COUNTER PAIN RELIEF GUM GEL.	I WOULD LIKE TO VISIT THE DENTIST.

~NOSE~

I DO NOT SEE A PHRASE I CAN USE.

LET'S USE THE ALPHABET CHART.	LET'S USE THE TOPICS CHART.

MY NOSE ITCHES.	THE INSIDE OF MY NOSE • BURNS • HURTS	MY NOSE IS STUFFY.
I THINK I HAVE A NOSE HAIR ITCHING THE INSIDE OF MY NOSE.	I HAVE A SORE IN MY NOSE.	I NEED TO BLOW MY NOSE.
	I NEED MY INHALER.	I NEED MY NASAL SPRAY.

~NECK ~

I DO NOT SEE A PHRASE I CAN USE.		
LET'S USE THE ALPHABET CHART.	**LET'S USE THE TOPICS CHART.**	
THE BACK OF MY NECK HURTS.	MY THROAT HURTS.	I HAVE BEEN COUGHING ALL NIGHT.
I SLEPT WRONG AND MY NECK HURTS.	THE GLANDS IN MY NECK FEEL SWOLLEN.	MY THROAT FEELS SWOLLEN.
MY NECK ALWAYS HURTS.	I WOULD LIKE THE BACK OF MY NECK MASSAGED.	I WOULD LIKE TO SEE MY DOCTOR.
I FEEL PRESSURE IN THE BACK OF MY NECK.		

~ARMS~

I DO NOT SEE A PHRASE I CAN USE.

LET'S USE THE ALPHABET CHART.	LET'S USE THE TOPICS CHART.

I HAVE PAIN IN THE

- RIGHT ARM
- LEFT ARM
- BOTH ARMS
- RIGHT ELBOW
- LEFT ELBOW
- BOTH ELBOWS
- LEFT SHOULDER
- RIGHT SHOULDER

I HAVE A BURNING SENSATION IN

- BOTH ARMS
- MY RIGHT ARM
- MY LEFT ARM

I HAVE A NUMBING FEELING IN

- BOTH ARMS
- MY RIGHT ARM
- MY LEFT ARM

~ARMS~

I DO NOT SEE A PHRASE I CAN USE.	
LET'S USE THE ALPHABET CHART.	LET'S USE THE TOPICS CHART.

I HAVE A TINGLING SENSATION IN

- MY RIGHT ARM
- MY LEFT ARM
- BOTH OF MY ARMS

IT FEELS LIKE I HAVE A PULLED MUSCLE IN

- MY RIGHT ARM
- MY LEFT ARM
- BOTH OF MY ARMS

I AM ITCHY ALL OVER

- MY RIGHT ARM
- MY LEFT ARM
- BOTH ARMS

~HANDS & WRISTS~

I DO NOT SEE A PHRASE I CAN USE.

LET'S USE THE ALPHABET CHART.	LET'S USE THE TOPICS CHART.

I HAVE PAIN IN

- MY RIGHT WRIST
- MY RIGHT HAND
- MY LEFT WRIST
- MY LEFT HAND
- BOTH WRISTS
- BOTH HANDS

ONE OF MY FINGERS HURT IN MY

- RIGHT HAND
- LEFT HAND

SEVERAL FINGERS HURT IN MY

- RIGHT HAND
- LEFT HAND

MY FINGERS ARE STIFF IN

- MY RIGHT HAND
- MY LEFT HAND
- BOTH HANDS

~ABDOMEN~

I DO NOT SEE A PHRASE I CAN USE.

LET'S USE THE ALPHABET CHART.	LET'S USE THE TOPICS CHART.

I HAVE AN UPSET STOMACH.

I FEEL NAUSEATED.

I AM HAVING ABDOMINAL CRAMPS.

I AM HAVING SHARP PAINS IN MY ABDOMEN ON THE

- RIGHT SIDE

- LEFT SIDE

- BOTH SIDES

I VOMITED ONCE.

I VOMITED SEVERAL TIMES.

I AM NOT HUNGRY.

I AM HAVING PAINS IN MY CHEST.

I AM HUNGRY.

I HAVE A RASH ON MY ABDOMEN.

~BACK~

I DO NOT SEE A PHRASE I CAN USE.		
LET'S USE THE ALPHABET CHART.		LET'S USE THE TOPICS CHART.
MY LOWER BACK HURTS.	IT FEELS LIKE I PULLED A MUSCLE IN MY BACK.	MY BACK ITCHES.
MY UPPER BACK HURTS.	I WOULD LIKE AN ICE PACK ON MY BACK.	PLEASE USE A BACK SCRATCHER ON MY BACK.
I WOULD LIKE A BACK MASSAGE.	I WOULD LIKE A HEATING PAD ON MY BACK.	I AM HAVING HEAT SENSATIONS ON MY BACK.

~BREASTS~

I DO NOT SEE A PHRASE I CAN USE.	
LET'S USE THE ALPHABET CHART.	LET'S USE THE TOPICS CHART.

I HAVE PAIN IN

- MY RIGHT BREAST

- MY LEFT BREAST

- BOTH BREASTS

I AM ITCHY AROUND MY BREASTS AREA.

I THINK I HAVE A RASH.

I WOULD LIKE THE CAREGIVER/NURSE TO EXAMINE ME.

MY BRA IS TOO

- LOOSE

- TIGHT

I HAVE A BURNING SENSATION IN

- MY RIGHT BREAST

- MY LEFT BREAST

- BOTH BREASTS

I WANT TO MAKE AN APPOINTMENT WITH MY GYNECOLOGIST.

I WOULD LIKE TO HAVE A MAMMOGRAM.

~BUTTOCKS~

I DO NOT SEE A PHRASE I CAN USE.	
LET'S USE THE ALPHABET CHART.	LET'S USE THE TOPICS CHART.

I THINK I HAVE A RASH ON MY BUTTOCKS.	IT HURTS WHEN I SIT DOWN.	I FEEL A • BURNING PAIN • SHOOTING PAIN • THROBBING PAIN
I NEED A NURSE TO EXAMINE ME TO SEE IF I HAVE A RASH.	I WOULD LIKE SOME POWDER FOR THE ITCH.	

~LEGS~

I DO NOT SEE A PHRASE I CAN USE.

LET'S USE THE ALPHABET CHART.	LET'S USE THE TOPICS CHART.

MY LEFT HIP HURTS.

MY RIGHT HIP HURTS.

BOTH OF MY HIPS HURT.

MY LEGS FEEL WEAK.

I HAVE PAIN IN

- MY RIGHT KNEE

- MY
- LEFT KNEE

- BOTH KNEES

I HAVE SHARP PAINS IN

- MY RIGHT LEG

- MY LEFT LEG

- BOTH LEGS

~LEGS~

I DO NOT SEE A PHRASE I CAN USE.

LET'S USE THE ALPHABET CHART.	LET'S USE THE TOPICS CHART.

THERE IS A TINGLING SENSATION IN	I HAVE A RASH ON	THERE IS A BURNING SENSATION IN
• MY RIGHT LEG	• MY RIGHT LEG	• MY RIGHT LEG
• MY LEFT LEG	• MY LEFT LEG	• MY LEFT LEG
• BOTH LEGS	• BOTH LEGS	• BOTH LEGS

~LEGS~

I DO NOT SEE A PHRASE I CAN USE.

LET'S USE THE ALPHABET CHART.	LET'S USE THE TOPICS CHART.

I NEED AN APPOINTMENT WITH MY DOCTOR TO SEE IF I HAVE A VITAMIN DEFICIENCY WHICH MAY BE CAUSING THE MUSCLE CRAMPS.

I HAVE NUMBNESS IN

- MY RIGHT LEG

- MY LEFT LEG

- BOTH LEGS

IT FEELS LIKE I PULLED A MUSCLE IN

- MY RIGHT LEG

- MY LEFT LEG

- BOTH LEGS

I WOULD LIKE MY LEGS MASSAGED.

~ANKLE~

I DO NOT SEE A PHRASE I CAN USE.	
LET'S USE THE ALPHABET CHART.	LET'S USE THE TOPICS CHART.

I FEEL PAIN IN	I THINK I TWISTED	I FEEL NUMBNESS IN
• MY RIGHT ANKLE • MY LEFT ANKLE • BOTH ANKLES	• MY RIGHT ANKLE • MY LEFT ANKLE • BOTH ANKLES	• MY RIGHT ANKLE • MY LEFT ANKLE • BOTH ANKLES
I WOULD LIKE A HEATING PAD FOR	I HAVE SWELLING IN	I WOULD LIKE AN ICE BAG FOR
• MY RIGHT ANKLE • MY LEFT ANKLE • BOTH ANKLES	• MY RIGHT ANKLE • MY LEFT ANKLE • BOTH ANKLES	• MY RIGHT ANKLE • MY LEFT ANKLE • BOTH ANKLES

~FEET~

I DO NOT SEE A PHRASE I CAN USE.

LET'S USE THE ALPHABET CHART.	LET'S USE THE TOPICS CHART.

I HAVE SHARP PAINS IN

- MY RIGHT FOOT
- MY LEFT FOOT
- BOTH FEET

I HAVE A TINGLING SENSATION IN

- MY RIGHT FOOT
- MY LEFT FOOT
- BOTH OF MY FEET

I HAVE NUMBNESS IN

- MY RIGHT FOOT
- MY LEFT FOOT
- BOTH FEET

~FEET~

I DO NOT SEE A PHRASE I CAN USE.

LET'S USE THE ALPHABET CHART.	LET'S USE THE TOPICS CHART.

I HAVE A BURNING SENSATION IN

- MY RIGHT FOOT

- MY LEFT FOOT

- BOTH FEET

THERE IS A TOENAIL CAUSING PAIN IN MY

- RIGHT FOOT

- LEFT FOOT

I WOULD LIKE A

- FOOT MASSAGE

- PEDICURE

I WOULD LIKE TO MAKE AN APPOINTMENT WITH A PODIATRIST.

MY FEET FEEL DRY PLEASE PUT LOTION ON MY FEET.

~DIGESTIVE~

I DO NOT SEE A PHRASE I CAN USE.

LET'S USE THE ALPHABET CHART.

LET'S USE THE TOPICS CHART.

I DO NOT HAVE AN APPETITE.

I ALWAYS FEEL HUNGRY.

I HAVE ACID-REFLUX AFTER EATING.

I FEEL NAUSEATED AFTER I EAT.

I WAKE AT NIGHT FROM ACID-REFLUX.

I AM ALWAYS THIRSTY.

I AM HAVING PAINS IN MY ABDOMEN.

I FEEL BLOATED AND UNCOMFORTABLE.

~BOWEL & URINATION ISSUES~

I DO NOT SEE A PHRASE I CAN USE.	
LET'S USE THE ALPHABET CHART.	**LET'S USE THE TOPICS CHART.**

I FEEL CONSTIPATED.	**I THINK I NEED AN ENEMA.**	**IT BURNS WHEN I URINATE.**
I HAVE PAIN FROM HEMORRHOIDS.	**MY URINE LOOKS DARKER THAN NORMAL.**	**MY URINE HAS AN ODOR.**
I WOULD LIKE TO TAKE A LAXATIVE OR STOOL SOFTNER.	**I FEEL LIKE I HAVE TO URINATE ALL THE TIME. I NEED TO BE CHECK FOR A URINARY TRACK INFECTION.**	
	I HAVE LOOSE BOWELS. I WOULD LIKE TO TAKE SOMETHING TO FOR THIS ISSUE.	

~RESPIRATORY~

I DO NOT SEE A PHRASE I CAN USE.

LET'S USE THE ALPHABET CHART.	LET'S USE THE TOPICS CHART.

I HAVE SHORTNESS OF BREATH.

MY CHEST

- FEELS TIGHT
- FEELS HEAVY
- HURTS

I HAVE BEEN COUGHING ALL NIGHT.

I WOULD LIKE TO BE CHECKED FOR SLEEP APNEA.

I AM COUGHING-UP

- COLORED MUCUS
- BLOODY MUCUS

I WOULD LIKE TO SEE MY DOCTOR.

~FEMALE ISSUES~

I DO NOT SEE A PHRASE I CAN USE.

LET'S USE THE ALPHABET CHART.	LET'S USE THE TOPICS CHART.

I AM MENSTRUATING.

I NEED SANITARY PRODUCTS.

I THINK I MAY HAVE AN INFECTION AND I NEED TO SEE MY DOCTOR. MY SYMPTOMS ARE:

- ITCHING
- BURNING
- ODOR
- CONSTANT URGE TO URINATE

I HAVE CRAMPS.

I WOULD LIKE TO TAKE A

- IBUPROFEN
- ADVIL
- TYLENOL

I AM EXPERIENCING HOT-FLASHES.

I WOULD LIKE TO HAVE A HEATING PAD.

I NEED TO MAKE AN APPOINTMENT WITH MY GYNECOLOGIST.

~MALE ISSUES~

I DO NOT SEE A PHRASE I CAN USE.

LET'S USE THE ALPHABET CHART.

LET'S USE THE TOPICS CHART.

I AM FEELING PAIN WHEN I URINATE.

I AM HAVING A BURNING SENSATION WHEN I URINATE.

THE COLOR OF MY URINE IS DARKER THAN NORMAL.

I AM VERY ITCHY AND MAY HAVE A RASH.

I WOULD LIKE A NURSE TO EXAMINE ME.

I WOULD LIKE SOME MEDICATED POWDER FOR THE ITCH.

I WOULD LIKE TO SEE MY DOCTOR.

I WOULD LIKE TO SEE A UROLOGIST.

~EMOTIONAL HEALTH~

I DO NOT SEE A PHRASE I CAN USE.	
LET'S USE THE ALPHABET CHART.	LET'S USE THE TOPICS CHART.

I FEEL FINE.	I FEEL BAD.	I AM HAVING ANXIETY.	I AM FEELING DEPRESSED.
I DO NOT HAVE AN APPETITE.		I WOULD LIKE TO SEE A PSYCHIATRIST.	
I CANNOT SLEEP.		I WOULD LIKE TO SEE A COUNSELOR.	
I AM NOT SLEEPING THROUGH THE NIGHT.		MY THOUGHT PROCESS IS BECOMING CONFUSED WHEN LISTENING TO OTHERS SPEAK.	
I AM HAVING BAD DREAMS.		I AM HAVING HALLUCINATIONS.	

~MY MEDICATION REQUEST~

-COMMUNICATION WITH MY CAREGIVER/FAMILY-

I DO NOT SEE A PHRASE I CAN USE.

LET'S USE THE ALPHABET CHART.	LET'S USE THE TOPICS CHART.

PLEASE REVIEW MY ALLERGIES LISTED ON PAGE 92.

IT IS TIME FOR MY MEDICATIONS.

I WAS GIVEN MY MEDICATIONS.

PLEASE CHECK THE REFILLS ON MY MEDICATION LABELS.

I WOULD LIKE SOMETHING FOR MY HEADACHE /MIGRAINE-

- TYLENOL
- ADVIL
- IBUPROFEN
- ASPIRIN
- BC POWDER
- MIGRAINE PRESCRIPTION

MY PRESCRIPTIONS SHOULD BE READY AT THE PHARMACY.

I NEED TO TAKE ONE OF MY PAIN PILLS.

I WOULD LIKE TO VISIT MY DOCTOR TO REVIEW MY MEDICATIONS.

I DO NOT SEE A PHRASE I CAN USE.

LET'S USE THE ALPHABET CHART.	LET'S USE THE TOPICS CHART.

I WOULD LIKE TO SEE MY DOCTOR.	I WOULD LIKE TO SEE A NURSE.	I NEED TO GO TO THE EMERGENCY ROOM.
I WOULD LIKE TO FIND A NEW DOCTOR.	MY HEART RATE FEELS FAST- I WOULD LIKE TO SEE MY DOCTOR.	I THINK I AM EXPERIENCING A SIDE EFFECT FROM ONE OF MY MEDICATIONS AND WE NEED TO CALL MY DOCTOR.
I WOULD LIKE TO GET A SECOND OPINION.	I WOULD LIKE TO HAVE MY BLOOD PRESSURE CHECKED.	

I DO NOT SEE A PHRASE I CAN USE.

LET'S USE THE ALPHABET CHART.

LET'S USE THE TOPICS CHART.

I WOULD LIKE YOU TO REVIEW MY MEDICATIONS.

I WOULD LIKE A PRESCRIPTION TO MANAGE MY PAIN.

I AM EXPERIENCING SIDE EFFECTS FROM MY MEDICATIONS.

I WOULD LIKE A PRESCRIPTION FOR MY MIGRAINES.

THE PAIN PILLS YOU PRESCRIBED ARE TOO STRONG.

I WOULD LIKE TO TRY A DIFFERENT BRAND OF MEDICATION.

I WOULD LIKE A PRESCRIPTION SLEEP AID.

THE PAIN PILLS YOU PRESCRIBED ARE NOT STRONG ENOUGH.

I WOULD LIKE TO DISCUSS MY EMOTIONAL HEALTH- PLEASE TURN TO PAGE 31.

I DO NOT SEE A PHRASE I CAN USE.

| LET'S USE THE ALPHABET CHART. | LET'S USE THE TOPICS CHART. |

IS MY TREATMENT PLAN
THE MOST CURRENT TREATMENT
AVAILABLE FOR MY CONDITION?

| ARE THERE ANY MEDICAL TRIALS I CAN PARTICIPATE IN? | DO YOU THINK I SHOULD HAVE BLOOD TESTS? |

| WILL YOU BE CHANGING ANY OF MY PRESCRIPTIONS? | WHAT ARE THE RISKS WITH THIS TREATMENT? |

ARE THERE ANY SURGICAL PROCEDURES
TO IMPROVE OR EASE MY CONDITION?

| I AM HAVING MUSCLE SPASMS IN MY | I AM HAVING OTHER HEALTH ISSUES LET'S USE THE TOPICS CHART TO REVIEW ANATOMY TOPICS. |

- ARMS
- LEGS
- FACE

PLEASE REVIEW MY ALLERGIES
LISTED ON PAGE 92.

~PHYSICIAN VISIT~
~MY PHYSICIAN'S QUESTIONS/RESPONSES~

I DO NOT SEE A PHRASE I CAN USE.	
LET'S USE THE ALPHABET CHART.	LET'S USE THE TOPICS CHART.

YES	NO	I FEEL FINE.
I AGREE.	I DO NOT AGREE.	I HAVE NOT BEEN FEELING WELL.

I NEED SOME TIME TO THINK ABOUT EVERYTHINGWE HAVE DISCUSSED.	I FEEL PAIN THERE: 1-LOW 2-MEDIUM 3-HIGH
I WANT TO DISCUSS WITH MY FAMILY WHAT YOU HAVE DISCUSSED WITH ME.	I FEEL PAIN: 1-ON AND OFF 2-CONSTANTLY

~PERSONAL HYGIENE~

I DO NOT SEE A PHRASE I CAN USE.	
LET'S USE THE ALPHABET CHART.	LET'S USE THE TOPICS CHART.
I WOULD LIKE TO TAKE A • BATH • SHOWER I would like to check the water temperature before entering the water.	PLEASE • WASH MY HAIR • DO NOT WASH MY HAIR
	I WOULD LIKE TO SHAVE TODAY.
I WOULD LIKE MY TEETH BRUSHED.	I WOULD LIKE MY TEETH FLOSSED.
I WOULD LIKE MY DENTURES SANITIZED.	I WOULD LIKE TO RINSE WITH MOUTHWASH.
MY DENTURES FEEL LOOSE.	I WOULD LIKE A MANICURE.

37

I DO NOT SEE A PHRASE I CAN USE.	
LET'S USE THE ALPHABET CHART.	LET'S USE THE TOPICS CHART.
I WOULD LIKE TO GO TO THE HAIR SALON.	I WOULD LIKE TO GO TO THE BARBER SHOP.
I WOULD LIKE TO HAVE THE FOLLOWING SERVICES: • BRAIDS • COLOR • HIGHLIGHTS • MANICURE • NEW HAIR STYLE • PEDICURE • PERM • STRAIGHTENING • TRIM • WASH & STYLED	I WOULD LIKE THE BARBER TO GIVE ME A • GIVE ME A SHAVE • GROOM MY BEARD • GROOM MY MUSTACHE

I DO NOT SEE A PHRASE I CAN USE.		
LET'S USE THE ALPHABET CHART.		LET'S USE THE TOPICS CHART.
I WOULD LIKE TO CHANGE MY CLOTHES.		THIS OUTFIT IS NOT COMFORTABLE.
I WOULD LIKE TO WEAR CLOTHING IN THIS COLOR:		
WHITE	BLACK	PINK
BROWN	BEIGE	PURPLE
RED	BLUE	ORANGE
I WOULD LIKE TO WEAR SOMETHING FESTIVE CELEBRATING THE HOLIDAY.	YELLOW	GOLD
	GREEN	SILVER

I DO NOT SEE A PHRASE I CAN USE.

LET'S USE THE ALPHABET CHART.	LET'S USE THE TOPICS CHART.

MY UNDERGARMENTS FEEL DAMP.

I WOULD LIKE TO CHANGE MY UNDERGARMENTS.

MY BRA IS

- TOO TIGHT

- TOO LOOSE

I WOULD LIKE TO WEAR UNDERWEAR MADE OF:

- COTTON

- NYLON

- FLANNEL

I WOULD LIKE TO WEAR THIS TYPE OF BRA-

- SPORTS
- UNDERWIRE
- WITHOUT AN UNDERWIRE

I DO NOT WANT TO WEAR A BRA.

I DO NOT SEE A PHRASE I CAN USE.

LET'S USE THE ALPHABET CHART.	LET'S USE THE TOPICS CHART.

I WOULD LIKE TO CHANGE INTO MY NIGHT CLOTHES.

I WOULD LIKE TO WEAR DIFFERENT NIGHT CLOTHES.

I LIKE THOSE NIGHT CLOTHES.

I WOULD LIKE TO WEAR WARMER NIGHT CLOTHES.

I WOULD LIKE TO WEAR COOLER NIGHT CLOTHES.

I DO NOT LIKE THOSE NIGHT CLOTHES.

I DO NOT SEE A PHRASE I CAN USE.

LET'S USE THE ALPHABET CHART.

LET'S USE THE TOPICS CHART.

I WOULD LIKE TO WEAR MY SLIPPERS.	I WOULD LIKE TO WEAR SOCKS.	I WOULD LIKE TO WEAR MY ROBE.
PLEASE REMOVE MY SLIPPERS.	PLEASE REMOVE MY SOCKS.	PLEASE REMOVE MY ROBE.

I DO NOT SEE A PHRASE I CAN USE.	

LET'S USE THE ALPHABET CHART.	**LET'S USE THE TOPICS CHART.**

I WOULD LIKE TO CHANGE MY SHIRT.	**I WOULD LIKE TO WEAR A WARMER SHIRT.**	**I LIKE THAT SHIRT.**
PLEASE BRING A FEW SHIRTS FOR ME TO CHOOSE.	**I WOULD LIKE TO WEAR A COOLER SHIRT.**	**I DO NOT LIKE THAT SHIRT.**
	I NEED TO WEAR A DRESS SHIRT.	**I WOULD LIKE TO WEAR A SWEATER.**

I DO NOT SEE A PHRASE I CAN USE.

LET'S USE THE ALPHABET CHART.

LET'S USE THE TOPICS CHART.

I WOULD LIKE TO CHANGE MY PANTS.

PLEASE BRING A FEW

- PANTS
- SHORTS

FOR ME TO CHOOSE.

I WOULD LIKE TO WEAR:

- CASUAL PANTS
- DRESS PANTS
- JEANS
- SHORTS

I LIKE THOSE PANTS.

I DO NOT LIKE THOSE PANTS.

44

I DO NOT SEE A PHRASE I CAN USE.

LET'S USE THE ALPHABET CHART.

LET'S USE THE TOPICS CHART.

PLEASE BRING A FEW DRESSES FOR ME TO CHOOSE.

I WOULD LIKE TO WEAR A CASUAL DRESS.

I LIKE THAT DRESS.

I WOULD LIKE TO CHANGE MY DRESS.

I WOULD LIKE TO WEAR A FORMAL DRESS.

I DO NOT LIKE THAT DRESS.

I DO NOT SEE A PHRASE I CAN USE.

LET'S USE THE ALPHABET CHART.	LET'S USE THE TOPICS CHART.

PLEASE BRING A FEW SUITS FOR ME TO CHOOSE.	I LIKE THAT ONE.	PLEASE BRING A FEW TIES & BELTS FOR ME TO CHOOSE.
I WOULD LIKE TO CHANGE MY SUIT.	I DO NOT LIKE THAT ONE.	PLEASE BRING A FEW DRESS SHIRTS TO MATCH MY SUIT.

I DO NOT SEE A PHRASE I CAN USE.

LET'S USE THE ALPHABET CHART.

LET'S USE THE TOPICS CHART.

I WOULD LIKE TO WEAR:

- BOOTS
- DRESS SHOES
- FLIP FLOPS
- HEELS
- SANDALS
- SNEAKERS

I LIKE THOSE SHOES.

I DO NOT LIKE THOSE SHOES.

PLEASE BRING A DIFFERENT COLOR.

I WOULD LIKE TO WEAR

- COTTON SOCKS
- STOCKINGS
- NYLON SOCKS
- ANKLE SOCKS

PLEASE REMOVE MY SOCKS/ STOCKINGS.

PLEASE BRING A FEW PAIRS OF SHOES FOR ME TO CHOOSE.

I DO NOT SEE A PHRASE I CAN USE.		
LET'S USE THE ALPHABET CHART.	**LET'S USE THE TOPICS CHART.**	
I WOULD LIKE TO WEAR SOME JEWELRY.	**I LIKE THAT ONE.**	**I DO NOT LIKE THAT ONE.**
EARRINGS	**SUNGLASSES**	**WATCH**
BRACELET	**RING**	**I WOULD LIKE TO CHANGE MY** • **HANDBAG** • **WALLET**
PENDANT	**TOE RING**	
NECKLACE	**HAT**	**SCARF**

I DO NOT SEE A PHRASE I CAN USE.	
LET'S USE THE ALPHABET CHART.	LET'S USE THE TOPICS CHART.

I WOULD LIKE MY CLOTHES WASHED.	MY CLOTHES FEEL DAMP.	PLEASE IRON MY CLOTHES.
PLEASE WASH THE BATH TOWELS AND BED LINENS.	I HAVE ITEMS FOR THE DRY CLEANERS.	I THINK THE LAUNDRY DETERGENT IS IRRITATING MY SKIN. PLEASE USE A DIFFERENT LAUNDRY DETERGENT.

I DO NOT SEE A PHRASE I CAN USE.	
LET'S USE THE ALPHABET CHART.	LET'S USE THE TOPICS CHART.
I AM HAPPY WITH MY CAREGIVER/NURSE.	THE CAREGIVER/NURSE IS NOT TRANSFERRING ME WITH CARE.
I AM NOT HAPPY WITH THE CAREGIVER/NURSE.	AT MEALTIME THE CAREGIVER/NURSE IS • NOT PATIENT • NOT LETTING ME FINISH MY MEALS • NOT PREPARING HEALTHY MEALS
I WOULD LIKE A NEW CAREGIVER/NURSE.	THE CAREGIVER/NURSE IS NOT VERY ATTENTIVE.

I DO NOT SEE A PHRASE I CAN USE.	
LET'S USE THE ALPHABET CHART.	LET'S USE THE TOPICS CHART.
THE CAREGIVER/NURSE IS NOT CHANGING ME IN A TIMELY MANNER.	THE CAREGIVER/NURSE IS NOT BATHING ME ENOUGH DURING THE WEEK.
THE CAREGIVER/NURSE IS NOT TAKING PROPER CARE OF MY OVERALL HYGIENE.	I WOULD LIKE TO FILE A COMPLAINT WITH THE CAREGIVER/NURSE MANAGER.
MY CAREGIVER/NURSE IS NOT BEING KIND TO ME.	I WOULD LIKE TO TRANSFER TO A DIFFERENT ASSISTANT LIVING / REHABILITATION FACILITY.

I DO NOT SEE ANYTHING I LIKE.

PLEASE WRITE DOWN THE AVAILABLE FOOD ITEMS AND I WILL DECIDE.

LET'S USE THE ALPHABET CHART.

LET'S USE THE TOPICS CHART.

I WOULD LIKE A YOGURT.

I WOULD LIKE SCRAMBLED EGGS WITH:

- CHEESE
- TOMATO
- ONION
- GREEN PEPPER
- HAM
- TURKEY

TOAST WITH

- BUTTER
- JAM

I WOULD LIKE FRUIT.

I WOULD LIKE CEREAL.

I WOULD LIKE OATMEAL.

I WOULD LIKE A POACHED EGG.

I WOULD LIKE SUNNY-SIDE-UP EGGS.

I WOULD LIKE PANCAKES.

I WOULD LIKE WAFFLES.

I WOULD LIKE FRENCH TOAST.

I DO NOT SEE ANYTHING I LIKE.

PLEASE WRITE DOWN THE AVAILABLE
FOOD ITEMS AND I WILL DECIDE.

LET'S USE THE ALPHABET CHART.	LET'S USE THE TOPICS CHART.

CHICKEN

FISH

TUNA SALAD

PASTA

SMOOTHIE:

- BLUEBERRY

- CHOCOLATE

CHICKEN SALAD

SOUP

- CHICKEN NOODLE

- CHOWDER

- MIXED FRUIT

- STRAWBERRY

- VANILLA

- VEGGIE

SANDWICH

- HAM

- TURKEY

- ROAST BEEF

VEGGIE PLATE

FRUIT PLATE

SALAD WITH:

- RANCH
- ITALIAN
- OIL & VINEGAR

ENSURE / BOOST

- CHOCOLATE
- VANILLA
- STRAWBERRY

YOGURT

- VANILLA
- STRAWBERRY
- BLUEBERRY

I DO NOT SEE ANYTHING I LIKE.

PLEASE WRITE DOWN THE AVAILABLE
FOOD ITEMS AND I WILL DECIDE.

LET'S USE THE ALPHABET CHART.	LET'S USE THE TOPICS CHART.

WATER	COCONUT WATER	ALOE VERA WATER

WATER

- MILK
- SOY MILK
- ALMOND MILK
- ORANGE JUICE
- PEACH JUICE
- FRUIT PUNCH

WINE

- RED
- WHITE
- BEER
- MIXED DRINK

SODA

- COKE
- DIET COKE
- PEPSI
- DIET PEPSI
- SPRITE
- DIET SPRITE
- ORANGE
- CHERRY
- GRAPE

MILKSHAKE

- CHOCOLATE
- VANILLA
- STRAWBERRY

TEA

- HOT
- ICE
- SWEET
- UNSWEET
- GREEN

COFFEE

- BLACK
- SUGAR
- MILK
- FRENCH VANILLA
- HAZELNUT

54

I DO NOT SEE ANYTHING I LIKE.

PLEASE WRITE DOWN THE AVAILABLE
FOOD ITEMS AND I WILL DECIDE.

LET'S USE THE ALPHABET CHART.	LET'S USE THE TOPICS CHART.

YOGURT

- BLUEBERRY
- CHOCOLATE
- STRAWBERRY
- VANILLA

DANISH

DONUTS

FRUIT COCKTAIL

APPLESAUCE

BAGEL:

- CINNAMON RAISIN
- PLAIN
- ONION

BAGLE WITH:

- BUTTER
- CREAM CHEESE & CHIVE
- CREAM CHEESE
- PEANUT BUTTER

FRUIT

- APPLES
- BANANAS
- BLUEBERRIES
- CANTALOUPE
- GRAPES
- PEACHES
- PEARS
- STRAWBERRIES
- WATERMELON

I DO NOT SEE ANYTHING I LIKE.

PLEASE WRITE DOWN THE AVAILABLE
FOOD ITEMS AND I WILL DECIDE.

LET'S USE THE ALPHABET CHART.	LET'S USE THE TOPICS CHART.

CAKE

- CHOCOLATE
- YELLOW
- CHEESE

COOKIES

- CHOCOLATE CHIP
- PEANUT BUTTER
- SUGAR

SHAKE:

- BANANA
- CHOCOLATE
- STRAWBERRY
- VANILLA

PIE

- APPLE
- KEYLIME
- PUMPKIN

ICE CREAM

- CHOCOLATE
- STRAWBERRY
- VANILLA

JELLO

- CHERRY
- WITH FRUIT
- ORANGE
- STRAWBERRY

PUDDING

- CHOCOLATE
- VANILLA

56

I DO NOT SEE A PHRASE I CAN USE.

LET'S USE THE ALPHABET CHART.	LET'S USE THE TOPICS CHART.

I WANT TO MAKE AN APPOINTMENT WITH MY ATTORNEY.

I DO NOT HAVE A LAWYER.

I NEED TO HIRE A LAWYER.

I WOULD LIKE TO HIRE A NEW LAWYER.

I NEED TO UPDATE MY ESTATE AND REVIEW ALL OF MY LEGAL DOCUMENTS.

~LEGAL DOCUMENTS~

I DO NOT SEE A PHRASE I CAN USE.

LET'S USE THE ALPHABET CHART.	LET'S USE THE TOPICS CHART.

I NEED TO HAVE A LAWYER DEVISE A-

OR

UPDATE MY-

- WILL

- LIVING WILL

- LAST WILL & TESTAMENT

- POWER of ATTORNEY

- POWER of ATTORNEY FOR ASSET MANAGEMENT

- HEALTHCARE PROXY

- HIPAA RELEASE FORM

I NEED MY END-OF-YEAR FEDERAL TAX RETURN FILED.

I WILL NEED THE ALPHABET CHART TO CONVEY WHERE MY PAPERWORK IS FILED FOR MY TAXES.

~MY EMPLOYMENT~

I DO NOT SEE A PHRASE I CAN USE.	
LET'S USE THE ALPHABET CHART.	LET'S USE THE TOPICS CHART.

I NEED TO CONTACT MY EMPLOYER.	I NEED TO MEET WITH SOMEONE IN THE HUMAN RESOURCE DEPARTMENT.	PLEASE DEPOSIT MY PAYCHECK.
I NEED TO CONTACT ONE OF MY COWORKERS.		I NEED TO CHECK MY BANK ACCOUNT ONLINE FOR A DIRECT DEPOSIT.
I NEED TO FILE FOR DISABILITY BENEFITS • WITH MY EMPLOYER • WITH SOCIAL SECURITY	I NEED TO FILE FORMS FOR A MEDICAL LEAVE.	I WILL NOT BE RETURNING TO WORK AND I NEED TO INFORM MY EMPLOYER.

~MY SELF-EMPLOYMENT~

I DO NOT SEE A PHRASE I CAN USE.

LET'S USE THE ALPHABET CHART.	LET'S USE THE TOPICS CHART.

I NEED TO ASSIGN AN OPERATIONS MANAGER IN MY ABSENCE.	I NEED TO SEE ONE OF MY EMPLOYEES.	I NEED TO TRANSFER FUNDS TO MY BUSINESS ACCOUNT.
I NEED TO SEE MY • BUSINESS PARTNER • OFFICE MANAGER	I NEED A BUSINESS LETTER DRAFTED. LET'S USE THE ALPHABET CHART.	I NEED TO MEET WITH MY • BOOKKEEPER • CPA • INSURANCE AGENT
I DECIDED TO • SELL MY BUSINESS • CLOSE MY BUSINESS	I DECIDED TO LOOK FOR A BUSINESS PARTNER. I NEED TO FILE FOR SOCIAL SECURITY DISABILITY.	I NEED TO MEET WITH AN ATTORNEY REGARDING MY BUSINESS.

~BANKING~

I DO NOT SEE A PHRASE I CAN USE.

LET'S USE THE ALPHABET CHART.	LET'S USE THE TOPICS CHART.

I NEED TO REVIEW MY BANK ACCOUNT(s).

I NEED TO MEET WITH A

- BANK OFFICER
- BANK MANAGER

I NEED TO MAKE A

- DEPOSIT
- TRANSFER
- WITHDRAWAL

I WOULD LIKE TO

- ADD AN ADDITIONAL SIGNER
- ASSIGN BENEFICIARIES
- OPEN A NEW ACCOUNT
- CLOSE MY BANK ACCOUNT(s)
- RENT A SAFETY DEPOSIT BOX
- CLOSE MY SAFETY DEPOSIT BOX

~HOME RESPONSIBILITIES~

I DO NOT SEE A PHRASE I CAN USE.

LET'S USE THE ALPHABET CHART.	LET'S USE THE TOPICS CHART.

I NEED TO
SEE MY-

- HUSBAND
- WIFE
- PARTNER
- MOTHER
- MOTHER-IN-LAW
- FATHER
- FATHER-IN-LAW
- MY SON
- SON-IN-LAW
- MY DAUGHTER
- DAUGHTER-IN-LAW
- SISTER
- SISTER-IN-LAW
- BROTHER
- BROTHER-IN-LAW
- RELATIVE
- ROOMMATE
- FRIEND
- PERSONAL REPRESENTATIVE

I NEED TO HIRE A YARD SERVICE.	I NEED MY HOUSE KEYS.
I NEED TO HIRE A POOL SERVICE.	I NEED AN EXTRA HOUSE KEY MADE.
I NEED MY NEWSPAPER CANCELLED.	I NEED MY MAIL BROUGHT TO ME.
	I NEED TO HAVE MY MAIL FORWARDED.

I NEED TO HAVE MY PET FOSTERED
UNTIL I AM WELL.
LET'S USE THE ALPHABET CHART
FOR ME TO CONVEY THE NAME OF THE
VETERINARIAN CLINIC WITH
ALL OF MY PET'S INFORMATION.

I WOULD LIKE TO ASK SOMEONE
I KNOW TO FOSTER MY PET(s).
PLEASE SHOW ME THE NAMES
LISTED ON PAGES 80-88.

~BILLS TO PAY~

I DO NOT SEE A PHRASE I CAN USE.		
LET'S USE THE ALPHABET CHART.		LET'S USE THE TOPICS CHART.
MORTGAGE /RENT	HOUSE ALARM	POOL SERVICE
HEALTH & DENTAL INSURANCE	LIGHT & WATER	
	LAWN SERVICE	
	CAR PAYMENT	BOAT PAYMENT
LIFE POLICY	CAR INSURANCE	BOAT INSURANCE
DISABILITY POLICY	CABLE / INTERNET	HOA FEES: • MONTHLY • QUARTERLY
CREDIT CARDS- I NEED TO REVIEW ALL ACCOUNTS.	HOME INSURANCE & PROPERTY TAX	I HAVE OTHER BILLS NOT LISTED. LET'S USE THE ALPHABET CHART.
PLEASE WRITE DOWN A LIST OF THE BILLS DUE.		

I DO NOT SEE A PHRASE I CAN USE.

LET'S USE THE ALPHABET CHART.	LET'S USE THE TOPICS CHART.

MY CAR IS LEASED
AND
NEEDS TO BE RETURNED.

I WANT TO GIVE MY CAR TO SOMEONE.	I WANT TO GIVE MY BOAT TO SOMEONE.
I WANT TO SELL MY CAR.	I WANT TO SELL MY BOAT.

I NEED SOMEONE TO SEARCH FOR THE TITLE(s)
FOR MY CAR(s) and or BOAT(s).
LET'S USE THE ALPHABET CHART FOR ME
COMMUNICATE WHERE I KEEP THE TITLES.

~ADDITIONAL ASSETS~

LET'S USE THE ALPHABET CHART.	LET'S USE THE NUMERIC CHART.	LET'S USE THE TOPICS CHART.
<u>ASSET NAME</u> & <u>ACCOUNT NUMBER</u>	IT HAS A MONTHLY PAYMENT.	OTHER

~FINANCIAL ASSETS~

I DO NOT SEE A PHRASE I CAN USE.	
LET'S USE THE ALPHABET CHART.	LET'S USE THE TOPICS CHART.

I NEED TO MEET WITH AN ATTORNEY.	I WANT TO SELL MY INVESTMENT PROPERTIES.	I NEED TO SEE MY FINANCIAL ADVISOR.
I NEED TO ASSIGN A POWER-OF-ATTORNEY TO HANDLE MY FINANCIAL PORTFOLIO.	I NEED TO CHANGE THE BENEFICIARIES ON MY: • LIFE POLICIES • BANK ACCOUNTS • OTHER ACCOUNTS	I WANT TO SELL MY: • STOCKS • ANNUITIES • OTHER

~ADDITIONAL FINANCIAL ASSETS~
~TO BE ADDRESSED~

ASSET	DESCRIPTION/INSTRUCTIONS
LET'S USE THE ALPHABET CHART.	LET'S USE THE NUMERIC CHART.

~MY ELECTRONIC DEVICES~

I DO NOT SEE A PHRASE I CAN USE.

LET'S USE THE ALPHABET CHART.	LET'S USE THE TOPICS CHART.

I WOULD LIKE YOU TO LOOK THROUGH THE CONTACTS IN MY CELL PHONE • CHECK MY EMAILS • TEXT MESSAGES	I NEED MY LAPTOP. • I WOULD LIKE YOU TO CHECK MY EMAIL • LOOK FOR A FILE STORED ON MY COMPUTER	I WOULD LIKE TO LISTEN TO MUSIC. PLEASE BRING MY • CELL PHONE • IPAD • LAPTOP • NETBOOK I WILL ALSO NEED MY HEADSET / EAR BUDS.
MY CELL PHONE HAS A PASSWORD. WE NEED TO USE THE ALPHABET & NUMERIC CHART TO CONVEY PASSCODE.	MY LAPTOP HAS A PASSWORD. WE NEED TO USE THE ALPHABET & NUMERIC CHART TO CONVEY PASSCODE.	MY IPAD/ NETBOOK HAS A PASSWORD. WE NEED TO USE THE ALPHABET & NUMERIC CHART TO CONVEY PASSCODE.

Passcode Reminder: If a passcode letter is signaled, ask if it is upper or lower case. Also, remember to ask if there is a dot (.) or underscore(_) between the screen names.

I DO NOT SEE A PHRASE I CAN USE.

LET'S USE THE ALPHABET CHART.	LET'S USE THE TOPICS CHART.

PLEASE TURN-ON THE TELEVISION.	PLEASE TURN THE VOLUME UP.
PLEASE TURN-OFF THE TELEVISION.	PLEASE TURN THE VOLUME DOWN.

PLEASE BROWSE THE CABLE CHANNELS.

PLEASE SEARCH FOR A MOVIE ABOUT:

- ACTION
- ADVENTURE
- CLASSIC
- COMEDY
- CRIME
- HORROR
- MYSTERY
- PSYCHOLOGICAL THRILLER
- RELIGIOUS
- ROMANCE
- SCIENCE FICTION
- SPORTS
- WAR
- WESTERN

PLEASE FIND A SHOW WITH:

- COMEDY
- CRIME INVESTIGATIONS
- DOCUMENTARY
- ENTERTAINMENT NEWS
- GAME SHOW
- INVESTMENT SHOWS
- LOCAL NEWS

- NATIONAL NEWS
- POLICE SHOWS
- POLITICAL SHOWS
- REALITY SHOW
- RELIGIOUS PROGRAM
- SOAP OPERA
- STAND-UP COMEDY
- TALENT SHOW
- TALK SHOWS
- WORLD NEWS

~MY WEEKLY TELEVISION FAVORITES~

SUNDAY				
MONDAY				
TUESDAY				
WEDNESDAY				
THURSDAY				
FRIDAY				
SATURDAY				

I DO NOT SEE A PHRASE I CAN USE.

LET'S USE THE ALPHABET CHART.

LET'S USE THE TOPICS CHART.

I WOULD LIKE TO GO OUT FOR

- BREAKFAST
- LUNCH
- DINNER
- DESSERT

PLEASE WRITE DOWN A FEW RESTAURANT CHOICES FOR ME TO CHOOSE.

I WOULD LIKE TO MAKE PLANS FOR

- MY BIRTHDAY

- THE HOLIDAY

- A PARTY

I WOULD LIKE TO GO

- FOR A DRIVE
- TO A CONCERT
- TO A PARK
- TO A PLAY
- TO A MOVIE
- TO A MUSEUM

~ENTERTAINMENT~

I DO NOT SEE A PHRASE I CAN USE.

LET'S USE THE
ALPHABET CHART.

LET'S USE THE
TOPICS CHART.

I WOULD LIKE
TO GO SHOPPING
AT THE

- GROCERY STORE
- MALL

DON'T FORGET TO BRING THIS
BOOK IN ORDER TO USE
THE SHOPPING CHART PAGE 96.

I WOULD LIKE
TO MAKE
PLANS FOR A

- DAY TRIP
- ROAD TRIP
- THEME PARK
- WEEKEND GETAWAY
- VACATION

I HAVE A SPECIAL DESTINATION REQUEST.
~LET'S USE THE ALPHABET CHART~

I DO NOT SEE A PHRASE I CAN USE.

LET'S USE THE ALPHABET CHART.	LET'S USE THE TOPICS CHART.

I WOULD LIKE TO SEE

- ONE OF MY CHILDREN
- MY DAUGHTER
- MY DAUGHTER-IN-LAW
- MY SON
- MY SON-IN-LAW

- ONE OF MY GRANDCHILDREN
- MY GRANDDAUGHTER
- MY GRANDSON

- MY MOTHER
- MY GRANDMOTHER
- MY FATHER
- MY GRANDFATHER
- MY PARENTS
- MY GRANDPARENTS

- MY BROTHER
- BROTHER-IN-LAW
- MY SISTER
- SISTER-IN-LAW

- ONE OF MY RELATIVES
- ONE OF MY FRIENDS
- ONE OF MY COWORKERS
- ONE OF MY EMPLOYEES
- MY PET

~SOCIAL COMMUNICATION~
-MY QUESTIONS FOR GUESTS-

I DO NOT SEE A PHRASE I CAN USE.		
LET'S USE THE ALPHABET CHART.		LET'S USE THE TOPICS CHART.
HOW ARE YOU?	HOW IS WORK?	ARE YOU PLAYING ANY SPORTS?
WHAT HAVE YOU BEEN DOING?	HOW IS SCHOOL?	WHAT DO YOU DO IN YOUR SPARE TIME?
WHAT DID YOU DO LAST WEEKEND?	WHEN DO YOU GRADUATE?	WHEN DID YOU GRADUATE?

~SOCIAL COMMUNICATION~
~MY QUESTIONS FOR GUESTS~

I DO NOT SEE A PHRASE I CAN USE.			
LET'S USE THE ALPHABET CHART.		LET'S USE THE TOPICS CHART.	
HOW IS YOUR PARTNER?	HOW IS YOUR FAMILY?	HOW ARE YOUR PARENTS?	HOW ARE YOUR GRAND-CHILDREN?
HOW IS YOUR HUSBAND?	HOW ARE YOUR CHILDREN?	HOW IS YOUR DAD?	HOW IS YOUR DOG?
HOW IS YOUR WIFE?	HOW ARE YOUR SIBLINGS?	HOW IS YOUR MOM?	HOW IS YOUR CAT?

~SOCIAL COMMUNICATION~
-MY RESPONSES-

I DO NOT SEE A PHRASE I CAN USE.		
LET'S USE THE ALPHABET CHART.		**LET'S USE THE TOPICS CHART.**
YES	I DO NOT KNOW.	I DO NOT UNDERSTAND.
NO	THAT IS HORRIBLE!	THAT IS WONDERFUL!
MAYBE	I LIKE THAT.	I DO NOT LIKE THAT.
I AM HAPPY!	I LOVE YOU!	I AM SAD.
I AM EXCITED!	I AM DISAPPOINTED.	I AM ANGRY!
I AM GLAD TO SEE YOU!		I AM HAPPY FOR YOU!
I DO NOT FEEL WELL TODAY.		I FEEL GREAT TODAY!

~SOCIAL COMMUNICATION~
-MY RESPONSES-

I DO NOT SEE A PHRASE I CAN USE.	
LET'S USE THE ALPHABET CHART.	LET'S USE THE TOPICS CHART.

I WOULD LIKE TO LEAVE.	I WOULD LIKE TO GO OUTSIDE.	I WOULD LIKE YOU TO CALL ONE OF MY CHILDREN.
I DO NOT WANT TO LEAVE.	I WOULD LIKE TO GO INSIDE.	I WOULD LIKE YOU TO CALL ONE OF MY GRAND-CHILDREN.
I RATHER STAY HERE.	I WOULD LIKE TO BE ALONE.	I WOULD LIKE YOU TO CALL ONE OF MY FRIENDS.
PLEASE HAVE A SEAT.	I ENJOYED YOUR VISIT.	I WOULD LIKE YOU TO CALL ONE OF MY FAMILY MEMBERS.

~PARTNER/SPOUSE TOPICS OF DISCUSSION~

- MEDICAL/DENTAL ISSUES
- HEALTH/DENTAL INSURANCE BENEFITS
- CAREGIVER ISSUES

- BILLS
- CAR ISSUES
- ESTATE PLANNING
- FINANCIAL ISSUES
- HOUSE ISSUES
- PREARRANGED FUNERAL PLANS
- RETIREMENT

- BIRTHDAY PLANS
- ENTERTAINMENT
- HOLIDAY PLANS
- VACATION PLANS

- MARITAL ISSUES
- RELIGIOUS ISSUES/SCHEDULES
- FUTURE PLANS
- JOB RELATED ISSUES
- RELOCATION

- CHILDREN
- CHILDREN'S EDUCATION
- CHILDREN'S FRIENDS
- GRANDCHILDREN
- FAMILY
- FRIENDS
- HUSBAND'S FAMILY
- WIFE'S FAMILY
- PETS

- AFTERNOON PLANS
- EVENING PLANS
- MORNING PLANS
- WEEKEND PLANS
- WEEK'S SCHEDULE

- DATE NIGHT
- ANNIVERSARY
- UPCOMING EVENT

- COUPLE COUNSELING
- FAMILY COUNSELING

LET'S USE THE ALPHABET CHART

LET'S USE THE TOPICS CHART

~SPOUSE/PARTNER COMMUNICATION~
~MY QUESTIONS & RESPONSES~

I DO NOT SEE A PHRASE I CAN USE.		
LET'S USE THE ALPHABET CHART.	LET'S USE THE TOPICS CHART.	

YES	YOU ARE WONDERFUL!	LET'S DISCUSS A DIFFERENT TOPIC.
NO	I LOVE YOU!	
MAYBE	THANK YOU!	
I WILL THINK ABOUT IT.	I FEEL GOOD.	I NEED THE PARTNER/SPOUSE TOPICS OF DISCUSSION AGAIN.
PLEASE DO NOT CHANGE THAT.	I AM NOT TIRED.	
WE NEED TO MAKE CHANGES.	I AM TIRED.	I DO NOT WANT TO DO THAT.
REVIEW THAT WITH ME.	GOODNIGHT!	I RATHER YOU NOT DO THAT.
LET'S GO OVER THIS LATER.	I AM UPSET WITH YOU.	I RATHER STAY HOME.
YOU SHOULD DO THAT.	I DO NOT FEEL WELL.	I WOULD LIKE TO DO THAT.

WHO?	WHAT?	HOW ARE THE KIDS DOING IN SCHOOL?	HAVE YOU TALKED TO THE TEACHER?
WHEN?	WHY?	HOW? DO THE KIDS HAVE ANY EVENTS THIS WEEKEND?	WHAT DO YOU THINK WE SHOULD DO?
HOW ARE YOU FEELING?		ARE YOU SIGNING THEM UP FOR ANY SPORTS?	ARE WE GOING TO MAKE PLANS?
ARE YOU GOING TO MAKE AN APPOINTMENT?		HAVE YOU MADE THEIR MEDICAL APPOINTMENTS?	WILL YOU PLEASE EXPLAIN THIS DECISION?

~NAMES OF MY GRANDCHILDREN~

~NAMES OF MY FRIENDS~

~NAMES OF MY FRIENDS~

~NAMES OF MY FRIENDS~

~NAMES OF MY EXTENDED FAMILY~

~NAMES OF MY EXTENDED FAMILY~

~NAMES OF MY COWORKERS~

~NAMES OF MY COWORKERS~

~ADDITIONAL CHARTS TO PERSONALIZE~

-YOU MAY WANT TO MAKE COPIES BEFORE COMPLETING-

I DO NOT SEE A PHRASE I CAN USE.		
LET'S USE THE ALPHABET CHART.		LET'S USE THE TOPICS CHART.

~ADDITIONAL CHARTS TO PERSONALIZE~

-YOU MAY WANT TO MAKE COPIES BEFORE COMPLETING-

I DO NOT SEE A PHRASE I CAN USE.		
LET'S USE THE ALPHABET CHART.		LET'S USE THE TOPICS CHART.

~ALPHABET CHART~

LET'S USE THE TOPIC CHART	**LET'S USE THE NUMERIC CHART**	

A	B	C	D	E	F	G
H	I	J	K	L	M	N
O	P	Q	R	S	T	U
V	W	X	Y	Z	SPACE	

~MY ALLERGIES~ TO FOODS & MEDICATIONS~

~YOU MAY WANT TO POST A COPY OF THIS ALLERGY LIST FOR AWARENESS~

FOOD ALLERGIES

NOTES:

MEDICAL ALLERGIES

NOTES:

~NUMERIC CHART~

| LET'S USE THE ALPHABET CHART | LET'S USE THE TOPICS CHART |

1	2	3	4	5
6	7	8	9	10
11	12	13	14	15
16	17	18	19	20
21	22	23	24	25
ADD	SUBTRACT	MULTIPLY	DIVIDE	EQUALS

I DO NOT SEE A PHRASE I CAN USE.

| LET'S USE THE ALPHABET CHART. | LET'S USE THE TOPICS CHART. |

I WOULD LIKE TO VISIT MY:

- CHURCH
- MONASTERY
- MOSQUE
- SYNAGOGUE
- TEMPLE

I WOULD LIKE RELIGIOUS COUNSELING.

~PLANNER TOPICS CHART~

I DO NOT SEE A PHRASE I CAN USE.	
LET'S USE THE ALPHABET CHART.	LET'S USE THE TOPICS CHART.

I WOULD LIKE TO GO OUT TODAY.	IS ANYONE COMING OVER TODAY?	IS ANYONE COMING OVER THIS WEEK?
<u>PHONE CALLS</u> I WOULD LIKE YOU TO CALL SOMEONE FOR ME-- LET'S LOOK AT THE NAMES CHART AND WORK WITH THE ALPHABET CHART TO CONVEY THE PHONE MESSAGE.	THIS WEEK I WOULD LIKE TO MAKE PLANS FOR A- • BREAKFAST OUT • LUNCH OUT • DINNER OUT • HAPPY HOUR • DATE NIGHT • GATHERING WITH FRIENDS • FAMILY NIGHT • DINNER PARTY	I NEED TO • PLAN OR • CHANGE MY PLANS FOR: • HOLIDAYS • BIRTHDAYS • EVENTS • MEDICAL APPOINTMENT • DENTAL APPOINTMENT • A PARTY • VACATION

LET'S REFER BACK TO THE ENTERTAINMENT
SECTION PAGES 71-72.

~SHOPPING CHART~I NEED TO BUY~

I DO NOT SEE A PHRASE I CAN USE.				
LET'S USE THE ALPHABET CHART.		LET'S USE THE TOPICS CHART.		
CLOTHES	SHOES	JEWELRY	MAKEUP	HYGIENE PRODUCTS
NIGHT CLOTHES	UNDER-GARMENTS	HAIR CARE PRODUCTS	EYE CARE PRODUCTS	SANITARY PRODUCTS
HOUSE ITEMS	FOOD ITEMS	SHEETS/ TOWELS	OVER-THE-COUNTER MEDICATIONS/ VITAMINS	MUSIC
AUDIO BOOK	MOVIES	GIFT CARD	A GIFT & GREETING CARD	MOVIE

~PERSONAL ITEMS REQUEST CHART~

PLEASE COMPLETE THIS CHART WITH
SPECIFIC ITEMS OWNED BY YOUR
FAMILY MEMBER / PATIENT.

~TOPICS CHART~

HEAD Pages 4-5	MALE ISSUES Page 30	ENTERTAINMENT Pages 71-72
EARS Page 6	EMOTIONAL HEALTH Page 31	PEOPLE I WOULD LIKE TO SEE Page 73
EYES Pages 7-8	MEDICATION & MEDICAL REQUESTS TO CAREGIVER Pages 32-33	SOCIAL COMMUNICATION MY QUESTIONS Pages 74-75
MOUTH Pages 9-10	PHYSICIAN VISITS Page 34-36	SOCIAL COMMUNICATION MY RESPONSES Pages 76-77
NOSE Page 11	PERSONAL HYGIENE Page 37-38	SPOUSE / PARTNER TOPICS CHART Pages 78-79
NECK Page 12	CLOTHING & LAUNDRY Page 39-49	FAMILY / FRIENDS NAME CARDS Pages 80-88
ARMS Pages 13-14	CAREGIVER ISSUES Page 50-51	ADDITIONAL BLANK CHARTS Page 89-90
HANDS / WRISTS Page 15	NUTRITION Pages 52-56	ALPHABET CHART Page 91
ABDOMEN Page 16	LEGAL ISSUES Pages 57-58	MY ALLERGIES Page 92
BACK Page 17	MY EMPLOYMENT Page 59	NUMERIC CHART Page 93
BREASTS Page 18	MY SELF-EMPLOYMENT Page 60	RELIGIOUS REQUEST Page 94
BUTTOCKS Page 19	BANKING Page 61	PLANNER TOPICS CHART Page 95
LEGS Pages 20-22	HOME RESPONSIBILITIES & BILLS Page 62-63	SHOPPING CHART Page 96
ANKLES Page 23	CAR & BOAT Page 64	MY PERSONAL ITEMS REQUEST CHART Page 97
FEET Pages 24-25	ADDITIONAL ASSETS Page 65	
DIGESTIVE Page 26	FINANCIAL ASSETS Page 66-67	
BOWEL & URINATION Page 27	MY ELECTRONIC DEVICES Page 68	
RESPIRATORY Page 28		
FEMALE ISSUES Page 29	TELEVISION Pages 69-70	